CHRISTMAS BASED GLUTEN-FREE RECIPES

Celina M. Moles

Copyright © 2022 by Celina M. Moles

All rights reserved.

No portion of this book may be reproduced in any form without written permission from the publisher or author, except as permitted by U.S. copyright law.

Contents

1. INTRODUCTION   1

2. TRADITIONAL BAKING   7

3. SUGAR GLAZE   29

4. ICING   31

5. GINGERBREAD LITTLE HUMANS   41

6. SPRITZ   45

7. LINZER COOKIES   49

8. GINGERBREAD FINGERS   59

9. NUTELLA COOKIES   63

10. CANDIED CHERRY AND WALNUTS   67

11. BISCOTTI WITH ALMONDS   71

12. PISTACHIO BISCOTTI   77

13. CAKE ICING   83

14. BRAZILIAN SWEETS   87

15. PEANUT BUTTER COOKIES   93

16. PINA COLADA OATMEAL COOKIES   97

17. CHOOLATE CHIPS COOKIES 101

18. CHOCO COOKIES FROM MEXICO 105

Chapter One

INTRODUCTION

Grain-Free, Pain-Free

People who can't tolerate gluten need to be aware of the dangers of not removing it from their diets, which is why gluten-free living is necessary. Gluten-free diets can alleviate terrible symptoms and suffering in as little as a few months, using food instead of medication. This is fantastic news. Those on a gluten-free diet don't have to give up their favorite baked products, including rich cakes, crispy cookies, and gooey pies, because there are plenty of options.

In order to keep us safe, our bodies have an intricate network of defenses. The immune system is a collection of organs, glands, and cell types that work together to protect the body from disease. There are situations when a poorly programmed immune system attacks healthy cells instead of potentially dangerous ones. Autoimmune illnesses are the medical term for these conditions.

2   CHRISTMAS BASED GLUTEN-FREE RECIPES

Numerous medical experts believe viruses that alter the information contained within cells are the most likely causes of autoimmunity illnesses, but there is still much to learn. The fact that far more women than males are affected by autoimmune illnesses suggests that sex hormones may possibly play a role.

Lupus, rheumatoid arthritis, and Graves' illness are all examples of autoimmune disease. Multiple sclerosis may also be triggered by an autoimmune reaction, according to some medical experts. Many of these diseases have complicated aggravating factors, but in the case of celiac disease, things are more simpler. Gluten, one of more than 30 proteins found in wheat, barley, and rye, is the trigger for celiac disease, which develops as a result of an immune system reaction.

The gluten protein cannot be adequately digested by humans as a species. Normally, protein is digested by the small intestine into minute particles known as amino acids, which are then utilized by the body as a source of sustenance. A lack of ability to effectively digest gluten appears to have no harmful impact on persons without gluten intolerance.

However, those who are sensitive to gluten are able to absorb the protein that isn't digested.

However, the small intestine does not recognize it as a source of sustenance. The body's immune system, on the other hand, views these protein particles as foreign invaders that must be eradicated, much like a virus, bacteria, or parasite. Inflammation and damage to the small intestine result, making it difficult for your body to absorb the nutrients it needs to function properly.

Normally, the small intestine is lined with tiny, hair-like projections called villi that resemble the deep pile of a plush carpet on a microscopic scale. Vitamins, minerals, and other nutrients are absorbed from the food you eat through villi in your digestive tract.

Without prominent villi, the inner surface of the small intestine becomes less like a soft carpet and more like a tile floor. The body is unable to absorb nutrients necessary for health and growth, leading in malnutrition.

The condition is much more widespread than previously thought, according to new research.

An estimated 1 in every 133 Americans has celiac disease, according to new research, making it one of the most common hereditary disorders in our country today. More than three million people are involved.

Anti-gliadin, anti-endomysial, and anti-tissue transglutaminase antibodies are used to diagnose gluten intolerance, which occurs when a person is exposed to gluten but disappears when the offending grains are no longer eaten.

4   CHRISTMAS BASED GLUTEN-FREE RECIPES

The gluten-free diet has helped millions of people with digestive issues who don't meet the formal diagnosis of celiac disease (because they don't test positive for the antibodies). Some 30 percent of Americans may fall under the category of gluten-sensitive, which is a better phrase than gluten-intolerant.

Gluten-free diets benefit a much broader range of people, allowing them to experience relief from everything from digestive problems to osteoporosis and nasal congestion. Psoriasis, anemia, and asthma have all been linked to gluten sensitivity.

You can't just go gluten-free and expect it to help your health.

It's a commitment that will last a lifetime. When gluten is eliminated from the diet, the body does not grow less susceptible to it.

When gluten is reintroduced into the diet, the problem will recur.

It's now easier than ever to eat a gluten-free diet thanks to the flood of gluten-free items flooding retailers. In normal supermarkets, rather than health food specialist shops, gluten-free ingredients for the delectable baked delights in this book may now be found. Because of these considerations, the recipes were created.

A lot of the ingredients featured in this book's recipes can be found in your kitchen pantry. Since the first time you made brownies as a kid, they've been a part of every cook's repertoire. This book is full with familiar ingredients, such as vanilla bean, eggs, and baking soda.

To add taste, you can add citrus and other fruits, such as tangerines and oranges, to the dough or batter. Crunchy nuts are used in some recipes, while sweet dried fruits are used in others. Cookies come in a variety of shapes and sizes, and they can either be rolled out and cut into creative shapes or cooked in a pan and sliced after they've cooled.

However, all-purpose flour, a vital component of traditional baking, is omitted from the list. And that omission causes a seismic shift in the political landscape. Neither wheat flour nor the gluten that is formed by two of wheat's intrinsic proteins can be substituted by any other granular substance.

Glucose is a wonderful substance. Crispy gingerbread people and chewy chocolate chip cookies are two of my favorite treats. This spectrum of textures has typically been achieved by the use of gluten.

More dry ingredients and a slightly different ratio of dry to wet ingredients are required for gluten-free baked goods to taste as excellent as those produced with wheat flour. In this chapter, you'll learn about the natural ingredients that go into baking delectable treats for your taste buds.

6   CHRISTMAS BASED GLUTEN-FREE RECIPES

Chapter Two

TRADITIONAL BAKING

When it comes to baked goods, science and art are given almost equal billing in the cooking process. There are certain hurdles to eliminating wheat from the diet, but eliminating all forms of wheat and wheat flour is a Herculean undertaking when it comes to baking. Baking relies on wheat flour, which has been a staple for millennia.

Proteins found in wheat flour (glutenin and gliadin) produce gluten when they're mixed with water. In order to generate elastic gluten strands, these two proteins bind with one another. To make the robust and bouncy gluten required for baking bread, flour with a high concentration of these proteins absorbs water more quickly. As in pie crust, the gluten generates tenderness when the proteins are covered with fat to make them shorter..

A recipe's elastic gluten network provides a variety of purposes. Gluten acts like a net, catching and retaining air bubbles. Baking soda or baking powder, for example, produce

8   CHRISTMAS BASED GLUTEN-FREE RECIPES

gas during the baking process, which causes the baked goods to rise and expand. As the oven heats up, moisture evaporates from the flour, resulting in the baked items' structure being set.

It's not an easy effort to replicate this structure. Wheat flour cannot be made gluten-free since the proteins are genetically encoded into the grain. A few other dry powders, though, can improve the outcome just as much.

Observing the Ingredients on Labels

Whenever you're looking for wheat on the ingredient labels, take caution! Wheat can be mentioned in a variety of ways, and it's often hidden. Bulgur is made from cracked wheat kernels, as are kamut and faro, two ancient varieties of wheat. Look for couscous as well, which is not a grain at all, but a granular pasta made from wheat flour. Semolina, farina, and durum wheat flour are all other names for the same thing. If you see one of these names on a product, it's gluten-free.

Wheat and Gluten-Free Grains and Flours

Unfortunately, when making gluten-free baked goods, there isn't a single ingredient that can replace all-purpose wheat flour 1:1. Even if the recipes appear lengthy because you need a lot of ingredients to produce the same texture as if you were using wheat flour, the ingredients are readily available even in most stores.

Finding wheat flour substitutes in the gluten-free baking aisle of supermarkets or searching online is a daunting task. As a bonus, several of these flours are significantly more nutritious than wheat.

In the gluten-free arsenal, each chemical has a unique set of characteristics. One will strengthen, another will tenderize, and a third will give moisture; all three are necessary for proper cooking. It's got all of these qualities in abundance.

Ingredients can be broken down into two main categories:

White and brown rice flour, for example, are high in protein and fiber, and as a result, these flours have a variety of beneficial properties. It isn't uncommon for cookies to be made with a combination of flavor and texture from flours in this category. But breads and other gluten-free meals should be made using them.

As a result, baked foods with soft crumb and a smooth texture can be produced by using starches, such as cornstarch, tapioca starch, potato starch, or sweet rice flour.

Baked foods created with protein/fiber flours are weighty and dense.

Baked items can't keep their shape if they're only made with starches.

10 CHRISTMAS BASED GLUTEN-FREE RECIPES

The key to successful gluten-free baking is to use a flour mix that includes both protein/fiber flours and starches. Baked items prepared with a wheat substitute can be just as tasty, if not better than those made with wheat.

Starches can be kept at room temperature, but flours should be refrigerated after opening. Refrigeration is the finest place to keep a pre-mixed baking mix if you have the space.

For ages, delicacies like classic French macarons have called for the use of almond meal, the only pre-packaged nut flour. A coffee grinder or mini-food processor works well for pulverizing blanched almonds. Peeled hazelnuts, for example, can be used as a substitute.

This flour is made from the tiny seed of amaranth, which was one of the main grains grown by the Aztecs. Lysine, an important amino acid, is substantially greater in this flour than in other grain flours. Complete proteins, like those found in meat and fowl, can be made by mixing amaranth with cornmeal.

The starchy flour prepared from the dried and ground roots of a tropical tuber, known as arrowroot, has two times the thickening ability of wheat flour and has no flavor at all. However, it can also be utilized in baked goods such as cookies and cakes.

a one-to-one substitution for cornstarch

In order to ensure that the cornmeal you purchase has not been contaminated with gluten, make sure you buy it from a reputable supplier. There are three types of cornmeal: fine-textured, medium-textured and coarse-textured.

Steel-ground corn is less nutritious than water- or stone-ground corn because less of the corn kernel is removed.

Arrowroot and cornstarch are the two most commonly used thickening agents in gluten-free cooking. In certain areas, it is referred to as corn flour, however this should not be mistaken with cornmeal. The endosperm of the corn kernel is ground into cornstarch after the kernels have been steeped for a few days, allowing the germ to be separated from the endosperm before grinding.

Potato Starch: Potato starch is distinct from potato flour, so be aware when you're purchasing it. Cooked potatoes are used to make potato flour, whereas raw potatoes provide the starch for the starch. In comparison to flour, which is much lighter in weight, the two can't be used interchangeably.

All-purpose wheat flour can often be replaced with rice flour, which has a mild flavor and can be used in a variety of recipes. Rice flour can be prepared from either white or brown rice, but the husk must be removed first. Because it contains some fiber, brown rice flour has a superior nutritional profile. The color of the baked cookie is the primary consideration when

12 CHRISTMAS BASED GLUTEN-FREE RECIPES

deciding which of these two ingredients to employ in a cookie recipe.

The Japanese term for sweet rice flour is "mochiko," and it may be found in Asian stores and supermarkets alike. To make cookie dough more flexible and sticky, it is created from glutinous short-grained Japanese rice. Tapioca starch is a good substitute for sweet rice flour if you don't have any on hand.

Cassava flour, or tapioca starch, is obtained from the tuber of the yucca plant, which is native to the tropics. In cookies, it provides structure and a chewy texture, and it aids in the browning of baked foods.

Oats, What About Them?

Recent research has convinced many groups that oats are safe to eat as part of a gluten-free diet. Despite the fact that oats are gluten-free, the difficulty is that they could be contaminated with

Gluten-containing grains are raised in the surrounding countryside. A majority of celiac groups in North America recommend oats that are not contaminated by other grains, and the packaging should indicate that the product is gluten-free or non-contaminated.

To use gums as a binding agent

TRADITIONAL BAKING   13

To ensure that the air introduced by yeast or chemical leavening agents is held until the proteins are cooked in the oven and form a structure, gluten gives cookie dough and batter its strength. Without the inclusion of natural gums, gluten-free flours and starches may not have the "stretch factor" needed to make cookies that aren't crumbly. In addition, they lend doughs and batters a tackiness of their own.

When using xanthan gum and guar gum, it is important to remember that they are two different powdered items that can be used interchangeably. They are included into the dry mix.

Xanthan gum, or corn sugar gum, is sometimes referred to as xanthan gum. It's a naturally occurring carbohydrate that doesn't get metabolized by the body and is therefore wasted. Xanthomonas campestris bacteria ferment the ingredients to create the additive. In the presence of corn sugar, this bacteria forms a white slime that is dried and processed to produce xanthan gum.

Most of Pakistan and northern India, where monsoons and droughts alternate often, are home to the guar plant, also known as the cluster plant. In some areas, guar is a significant cash crop. Harvested plants are left to dry out in the sun for a few days before being sold. Separation and processing of the seeds is next done manually or mechanically.

14 CHRISTMAS BASED GLUTEN-FREE RECIPES

It doesn't matter if you've eaten xanthan gum before, as long as it's on the label. A real food, not something made in a lab, is what it is. In order to prevent crystallization of sugar, manufacturers add xanthan gum to candies, as well as to many ice creams, in order to achieve a smooth texture and tongue feel.

Recipe Conversion and Basic Baking Ingredients

A baked good's flour and starch percentage is determined by the type of baked good you're creating. There is a vast variety of wheat flours to choose from when baking.

how it's put to use Bread flour, for example, has a high protein content because it is made from hard wheat, while cake flour has a low protein content because it is made from soft wheat.

In my opinion, making a customized mix for a specific baked good rather than using an all-purpose gluten-free baking blend would be preferable. This recipe is one I came up with that can be used in a one-to-one substitution for all-purpose wheat flour in many cookie recipes, from crunchy to chewy and light to dense. When adapting family recipes for gluten-free baking, use this formulation, but when using one of the recipes in this book, use the specific formulation provided with each recipe.

In addition to the xanthan gum, the base of my Basic Baking Mix contains rice flour.

TRADITIONAL BAKING 15

Rice flour can be replaced with up to a cup of almond meal for nut cookies.

Mixture for Making Simple Desserts

3 cups of liquid are produced.

Ingredients

rice flour, either white or brown, 2 cups

Sweet rice flour is 1/3 of a cup.

Potato starch is a third of a cup

Tapioca starch, one-third of a cup

Xanthan gum 2 teaspoons

Combine the ingredients in a bowl and chill in a container that can't leak.

Ingredients that may be helpful in the process

Aside from the dry ingredients, the recipes in this book make use of tried-and-true techniques for baking gluten-free.

As a replacement for the protein that gluten in wheat provides, eggs play an increasingly essential part in baking. They are a fantastic source of protein and help to give baked goods their structural integrity. While delivering protein, they also help starches to harden by releasing steam. The fat and lecithin in egg yolk make it an excellent source of emulsifying agents, which make it simpler to integrate air into doughs and batters.

16 CHRISTMAS BASED GLUTEN-FREE RECIPES

Sugar: Sugar enhances the sweetness of baked goods while also assisting in the browning process. When baking, sugar combines with egg protein and butter dairy proteins, resulting in browning, and the more sugar there is in the cookie dough, the more brown the finished product will be. Cookies may be kept fresher for longer because to the moisture-holding properties of sugar. Sugar crystals, along with solid fat, are responsible for creating small holes in the dough, which are then enlarged by leavening chemicals.

Today's commonplace granulated sugar was once so valuable and uncommon that it was dubbed "white gold." A perennial plant that originated in Asia but is now produced in nearly every tropical and subtropical region of the world, sugar cane is the primary source of sugar. Beet sugar refining only became regular practice in the nineteenth century.

Baked goods made with solid fats and crystalline sugar will have a fine and aerated texture because of the incorporation of microscopic air cells.

In addition to providing lubrication and a smooth taste, fat is also responsible for the luscious tongue feel. When it comes to baking, I exclusively use unsalted butter. Butter's milk fat gives baked goods their tenderness, color, and structure. In addition, it releases a mouthwatering aroma.

In baking, leavening agents include anything that causes baked goods to rise and foam. Because air is a natural leavener, many cookie dough recipes instruct bakers to beat the butter and sugar to a "light and fluffy" consistency. The added air is responsible for the puffiness and lightness of the finished product.

However, the majority of the time, baking soda and baking powder are used as the principal leavening agents. When they are mixed with water, both of these generate carbon dioxide. Sodium bicarbonate, or baking soda, must be used in conjunction with sodium bicarbonate.

baking powder is a mixture of baking soda and cream of tartar, both of which are acidic, and an acidic substance like buttermilk. baking powder and baking soda are interchangeable, despite the fact that baking soda is twice as potent.

Baking powder, on the other hand, should be examined carefully. Wheat starch is used as a "moisture absorption agent" by some brands. Rumford and Davis are two well-known companies that employ cornstarch and potato starch in their baking powder.

However, take sure to carefully read any labeling.

Chemical leavening isn't a new invention. Pearl ash was a literary device employed by Amelia Simmons in her novel.

1796 publication of American Cookery. A century ago, because the acid-base reaction releases carbon dioxide more quickly

18 CHRISTMAS BASED GLUTEN-FREE RECIPES

than does the fermentation process produced by living yeast, chemically leavened loaves became known as "quick breads."

Keep the Environment Clean

A newbie to gluten-free baking, or a person who must adhere to a strict gluten-free diet, may not be familiar with the concept of contamination. In the long run, it is worth the effort to create a system that prevents gluten-containing and gluten-free foods from coming into contact. To ensure that your gluten-free products are not contaminated by wheat flour or any other item containing gluten, here are some guidelines:

• Make sure everyone who uses the kitchen is aware that the cabinets where gluten-free food is stored are thoroughly cleaned. It is, nevertheless, a good idea to store gluten-free products in airtight containers before keeping them, unless the kitchen is completely devoid of gluten-containing meals.

• Before beginning to cook gluten-free dishes, thoroughly clean the kitchen surfaces and then change the dishrag and dishtowel for a new one. Don't use a sponge because it can't be washed thoroughly enough to remove gluten from it. Wooden cutting boards and other porous surfaces are the same. For gluten-free ingredients, have separate containers.

For gluten-free baking, keep separate containers of butter or margarine. Some breakfast butter may have come into contact with crumbs from a piece of toast that was eaten earlier that day.

Do not use the same sieve for gluten-free and conventional flour. Clearly label gluten-free products.

Avoid mistakes by using a free sifter.

• Store all ingredients for gluten-free baking in separate containers. Molecules of wheat flour could have settled on granulated sugar or baking soda, even though they do not contain gluten.

• When cooking gluten-free items, always place them on the highest shelf of the oven to reduce the chance of a spill. Similarly, gluten-free goods should be placed on the upper shelves of the refrigerator.

If you're concerned about contamination, use foil. When preparing, cooking, or storing food, use aluminum foil to keep items separate.

Stickers of different colors can be used to separate gluten-free goods from other foods when storing them.

Because it's not rocket science, baking may have been the first kitchen activity that most of us attempted as youngsters. It's important that you follow these tips to ensure that your baked goods are "smart cookies" every time.

20 CHRISTMAS BASED GLUTEN-FREE RECIPES

These are general ideas to help you with all your baking and cooking, not just gluten-free baking.

Basics of Baking

When it comes to baking, even if cooking is a sort of art, science also plays a role. Unlike savory recipes, which allow for an almost unlimited number of modifications, sweet recipes must be strictly adhered to. In a recipe, each ingredient has a distinct purpose based on the amount needed to make a batter or dough. Baked items of all kinds can benefit from these broad guidelines:

Ensure that your measurements are precise. Dry measuring cups, which are either plastic or metal and come in sizes of 1/4, 1/3, 1/2, 3/4, and 1 cup, are used to measure dry substances. In order to accurately measure dry ingredients, scoop them from the container or canister and sweep the top with a straight edge such as the back of a knife or spatula. Don't use the canister or the counter to make a flat surface by dipping or tapping the cup therein. The dry ingredients are compressed using these techniques, which can result in an increase in volume of up to ten times.

leveling is also required for tablespoons and teaspoons; a circular 1/2 teaspoon.

Nearly 1 teaspoon may be measured using this device. If the box or can doesn't have a built-in straight edge, use the

TRADITIONAL BAKING   21

back of a knife blade to level the spoon's surplus into the container. Liquid measures, which come in a variety of sizes but are made of clear glass or plastic, include lines on the sides for determining the volume of liquid. For accurate liquid measurements, put the cup on a flat surface and bend down to see the designated level at eye level.

Keep the temperature stable. Aside from the spices, all components should be at room temperature unless stated differently. Making a homogenous mixture is easier when all of the ingredients are at the same temperature. By making the fat more stiff, cold liquid can cause a dough or batter to lose its uniform structure.

• Start the oven. A temperature of 450°F may take up to 25 minutes to reach in some ovens. The heating duration should be no less than 15 minutes at a minimum.

• Be prepared. Assemble your ingredients and read the instructions attentively. All of the ingredients needed to make a recipe are pre-planned so you don't find yourself improvising at the last minute. The mixer will continue to run while you look for a specific spice or bag of chips if you put everything together ahead of time.

Creaming with Caution

The "creaming" of the butter and sugar is probably the most important phase in the making of a cookie dough. Air is incorporated into the butter's crystalline structure during this procedure. In order to leaven a dough or batter, the number and size of air bubbles (which are then increased by the carbon dioxide created by baking soda or baking powder) must be just right.

The temperature of the butter is the first step in good creaming, and it should be around 70 degrees Fahrenheit. Each stick of butter should be sliced into around 30 slices when it's out of the fridge. After allowing them to sit for 15 to 20 minutes at room temperature,

minutes to become pliable

Using a mixer, whip the butter into small pieces until it is no longer lumpy. Sugar is next added and mixed in at medium speed to begin the blending. Make sure you scrape your bowl periodically as you increase your machine's speed. The butter and sugar mixture will be light and fluffy once it has been properly creamed.

The 101st lesson in chocolate

High-quality chocolate is essential for any chocolate dishes' success. With the following exceptions, it is critical to use the type of chocolate stated in the recipe, as the amount of additional sugar and other ingredients is calculated based on the sweetness level. Using a different brand of chocolate could alter the flavor. After that, we'll get to the fun stuff. What you need to know about chocolate:

• No added sugars. This is the finest of all cooking chocolates, often known as baking or bitter chocolate. It is made from cocoa liquid that has been hardened and has no added sugar. It comes in bars of eight blocks each weighing one ounce. Unsweetened chocolate must comply with the American criterion of identification, which stipulates

cocoa butter content ranges from 50 to 58 percent.

Sweet but sour. The amount of sugar used to sweeten this chocolate differs from maker to manufacturer. If you want a really strong chocolate flavor, choose this chocolate, which should have at least 35% chocolate liquor in it. In baking and cooking, it can be used in place of semisweet chocolate.

• Slightly sweet. Unlike bittersweet chocolate, this chocolate is sweetened with sugar, but it can also be flavored with additional ingredients like vanilla. Bars, chips, and bits are all options.

Sweet food preparation This chocolate must contain at least 15% chocolate liquor, and it almost always has a higher sugar content than semisweet chocolate. Bars of four ounces are the most common size.

• Dairy products. To bake with this type of chocolate, you'll need to use a lot of milk chocolate chips. As little as 10%

24 CHRISTMAS BASED GLUTEN-FREE RECIPES

chocolate liquor can be used in this product, but it must also contain at least 12% milk solids.

• Cocoa powder without added sugar. Cocoa butter has been removed from this powdered chocolate. Cocoa keeps indefinitely in a cool area.

• Dutch-process cocoa powder. This sort of cocoa powder has a lower acidity level and provides a more mellow flavor to meals. Although it burns more slowly than regular chocolate, it also has a lower melting point.

Dark chocolate, like excellent wine, gets better with age. Store it in a cool, dry place. However, a gray "bloom" of chocolate has grown.

It's still safe to cook with, even though it was stored at a temperature that was too high.

How to Substitute with Confidence

Depending on your own preferences, you can use any combination of bittersweet, semisweet, or sweet chocolate in a recipe. It's better to go from a semisweet to a bittersweet chocolate rather than the other way around because most chocolate recipes tend to be sweet.

Chocolate chips and chunks of broken up chocolate should not be substituted for one another.

For high-heat baking, chocolate chips are designed to preserve their structure and behave differently than chopped chocolate does, which is why they're commonly used. Gritty grains can occur when chocolate chips have cooled down.

Take Caution When Working With This.

If you're going to eat chocolate out of your hand or fold it into cookie dough, you're going to have to be a little more careful. When it comes to frequent duties related with chocolate, follow these guidelines:

Chopping up chocolate. It's simpler to melt if you chop it up finely. In a food processor equipped with a steel blade, you can do this. Instead of shattering it with your hands, start by using a large knife. The chocolate will not be evenly chopped because of the heat generated by the body.

The chocolate is melting. To prevent scorching, most chocolate should be melted slowly and gently.

There are a variety of methods for melting it:

Chunks can be melted in a double boiler set on a low heat.

• In a microwave-safe bowl, place the chopped chocolate and microwave it on Medium (50%) for one minute.

30 seconds at 100 percent power. As needed, stir and re-stir.

26   CHRISTMAS BASED GLUTEN-FREE RECIPES

• Set the oven to 250°F. Turn on the oven and immediately remove the chopped chocolate from it. Return to the oven if necessary after 3 minutes of cooking.

There are a number of ways in which you can make chocolate smooth, but all of them need you to first melt the chocolate.

Drizzling the pan of bar cookies before cutting them into pieces is a simple technique to spruce up the desserts. Dip a spoon into the melted chocolate, then wave it over the cookie pan. You can also put the chocolate in a heavy-duty plastic bag and cut off the tip of one of the corners to make it easier to work with it.

Equipment That Matters

The following are some of the tools I relied on frequently when creating the recipes for this book:

Temperature gauge for deep-frying candy or deep-frying deep-frying. With the visual and textural signals I provide in Chapter 10, it is possible to take an accurate reading of the temperature of sugar syrup, which is essential to all candies and some cookies.

A microplane grater is also available. Basically, it looks like a flat kitchen spatula, except it has a few little holes in it.

You can use it to finely grate ginger and citrus zest.

TRADITIONAL BAKING   27

• A food processor. The food processor has its own section in my dishwasher because it is such an important piece of kitchen equipment. However, a second bowl can be purchased for very little money and used as a replacement for the base for creating gluten-free food. Plastic, the material used in food processors, can trap food particles if scratched.

• Cooling racks made of wire. These are absolutely necessary, and there is no substitute for them. An impermeable surface, such as the rack on a broiler pan, can make crispy cookies soggy faster than anything else. • A strong mixer, which will help the cookie dough come together more quickly. When the dough is particularly thick, a counter-top mixer is your best friend. Even while handheld mixers can be useful in some situations, a stand mixer is the ideal option for baking. Balloon whip attachments are great for making meringues, and paddles make the thickest substances look effortless to combine.

• Spatulas with offset blades. Transferring cookies from baking sheets to cooling racks is made simpler and more pleasant with this style of spatula, which has a handle elevated above the blade's level.

Creating a "Game Plan" for Cookies

Only once a year is it OK to create many cookie recipes per day during the holiday season. If you're going to be in the kitchen for a while, you'll want to create a lot of cookies. Don't,

28   CHRISTMAS BASED GLUTEN-FREE RECIPES

however, allow yourself to become paralyzed by fear. You can use this as a guide:

Make a pan of bar cookies to get things started; they go together quickly but take the longest to bake. For rolled cookies that require chilling before baking, the oven is now hot enough to begin making the doughs.

Make a batch of drop cookies as your third cookie type. Because these cookies don't require chilling time before baking, you may roll and cut out chilled dough while the bars are baking.

No need to ever leave the oven unattended when baking cookies from this book. Make the 375°F-baked batches last, because they take the longest to prepare.

There are, of course, meringues to round out the list. They are baked at the conclusion of the process because they are kept in a cool oven for a long period of time. But before you start baking again, make sure they're in the oven! Preheating the oven the next day to a high temperature has ruined many a batch that I forgot were still in there.

Developing the skills to become a Master Pastry Picasso

There are various recipes in Chapter 3 for decorated cookies, including icing-painted or candy-decorated ones. Learn how to decorate them both before and after baking in this section.

Chapter Three

SUGAR GLAZE

Glaze made from confectioners' sugar

Covering cooled cookies with this method is the most basic and takes less than an hour to harden.

1 and a half cups

5 minutes of active time

5 minutes from beginning to end

Ingredients

Confectioners' sugar in the amount of 4 cups

4 to 5 tbsp. of liquid

Clear vanilla extract is half a teaspoon.

Colored food dyes (optional)

First, whisk together 4 tablespoons of water and the vanilla extract in a mixing dish.

CHRISTMAS BASED GLUTEN-FREE RECIPES

Using extra water if necessary, stir until the mixture is smooth.

Add a few drops of food coloring at a time to the glaze until you achieve the desired hue. Before adding any extra coloring, mix thoroughly.

Remember that you can store the glaze for up to six hours at room temperature in an airtight container with plastic wrap immediately on the surface. Just a couple of quick beats will get it emulsified and ready for use.

Variations

Replace the water with orange juice and the vanilla extract with orange extract.

Vanilla can be replaced with peppermint oil or almond extract.

How to Make the Most of It

Confectioners' Sugar Glaze is not strong enough to hold large candies, but it can be used as "glue" for little objects like jimmies. White glaze can be applied on cookies that have cooled and hardened. Then, using food coloring, combine 1 teaspoon of water with 1/4 cup of glaze. Using a piece of waxed paper, crumple it up and dip it into the coloured glaze; then, using a pastry brush, apply a marbled appearance to the cookies.

Chapter Four

ICING

Icing with a royal touch

Once the cookies have cooled, the frosting can be applied with this recipe. Because it becomes sticky when chilled, this frosting should only be applied to cookies that have been kept at room temperature.

31/2 cups of food are produced with this recipe.

5 minutes of active time

12 minutes from the start to the end

Ingredients

At room temperature, three big egg whites.

0.5 tsp. cream of tartar

Salt with a quarter teaspoon

Confectioners' sugar in the amount of 4 cups

Vanilla extract in its purest form:

32 CHRISTMAS BASED GLUTEN-FREE RECIPES

Colored food dyes (optional)

Egg whites should be beaten until foamy with an electric mixer on medium speed, in a grease-free mixing dish. Using an electric mixer, whip the mixture on high speed until it forms soft peaks.

2. Add the sugar and beat on low speed to moisten the dough. Beat for five beats at a fast pace.

For up to seven minutes, or until the mixture is glossy and stiff peaks have formed. Add vanilla to the mix.

If you're coloring icing, start with a few drops of food coloring and work your way up to the desired shade. Before adding any extra coloring, mix thoroughly.

The frosting can be stored in an airtight jar at room temperature for up to 2 days.

days. Just a couple of quick beats will get it emulsified and ready for use.

Variations

Lemon or orange oil or almond extract can be used in place of vanilla if you choose.

How to Make the Most of It

ICING 33

This consistency of Royal Icing is ideal for decorating cooled cookies with piping and can also be used as a "glue" to attach candy. The cookies can be decorated with icing if desired.

In order to achieve the desired consistency, thin the icing with milk in 1-teaspoon increments until it reaches the desired consistency.

Using buttercream icing

Since this icing is produced with butter, it's not as white as Royal Icing, which is created with confectioners' sugar. It does harden a little, but not enough to form a genuine glaze.

Two and a half cups

5 minutes of active time

5 minutes from beginning to end

Ingredients

Softened unsalted butter, 1/4 pound (1 stick)

Confectioners' sugar in the amount of 4 cups

3 tbsp. of whole milk

1 tsp. of pure vanilla essence

Colored food dyes (optional)

34 CHRISTMAS BASED GLUTEN-FREE RECIPES

In a large mixing basin, combine the butter, sugar, milk, and vanilla extract. A low-speed electric mixer can be used to blend the ingredients. Beat on high for 2 minutes or until fluffy.

2. When tinting icing, divide the icing into small cups and add a few drops of food coloring at a time until you achieve the desired color. Before adding any extra coloring, mix thoroughly.

The frosting keeps well in the refrigerator for up to five days if stored in an airtight container. Before using, allow it to come to room temperature.

Variations

Vanilla can be replaced with almond extract, lemon oil, or orange oil.

How to Make the Most of It

Rosettes and other complicated embellishments can be made with buttercream using a pastry bag. Add confectioners' sugar in 1-tablespoon increments if necessary to get the desired stiffness..

Paint made with eggs

More intense colors can be achieved with beaten egg yolks and food coloring than with Royal Icing. It reminds me of the medieval European churches' tempera paintings.

Ingredients

ICING   35

Egg yolks from 4-5 eggs

Colored food dyes

Divide around 4 or 5 egg yolks into tiny cups by whisking them thoroughly.

2. Add food coloring at around the ratio of 1/2 teaspoon per egg yolk, and stir well.

Start by drawing a design on the cookies using the tip of a paring knife so that the colors don't mix.

Apply the color on the cookies before they are baked with a little paintbrush. In the oven, the colors will darken significantly.

Paintbrushes, on the other hand, are considerably less expensive than pastry brushes. A pastry brush can be made from any natural-bristle paintbrush.

Using Sweets and Candy

Colored and flavored sweets can be attached to cookies in an almost infinite number of ways. To apply some, you must do it before the cookies are baked, and for others, you must apply them after the cookies have cooled.

For the most part, hard and soft candy should be applied after cooking, whereas any candy that is primarily an ingredient like coarse colored sugars, gold or silver dragées, nuts, or candied fruit should be applied prior to baking. This is a general rule.

36   CHRISTMAS BASED GLUTEN-FREE RECIPES

Both ways can be utilized for ingredients like raisins. For gingerbread people and snowmen, the "eyes" should be placed before baking, but for wreaths, the decorations should be added after frosting.

Stencils can be used to create patterns using colored sugars after the cookies have been baked. When the cookie has cooled, spread either Royal Icing or Confectioners' Sugar Glaze on it, and then place a parchment paper stencil over it. Through the stencil's hole, add sugars or jimmies.

The term "Christmas cookie" conjures up images of buttery, crisp cookies in a variety of shapes and sizes, usually topped with a colorful frosting and sometimes some candies. There are other gingerbread men with little smiles and buttons down their "jackets" behind this image. As a bonus, you'll be pleased to learn that many of your favorite dishes can be made with gluten-free ingredients.

Due to the lack of gluten, it is necessary to make substitutions in order to achieve a stiff enough dough to roll. In order to properly chill the dough, it will take some time. This allows the butter to firm up again after it has been softened during the mixing process. Rolling the cookies thin enough to cut them out is a piece of cake after that.

For delicate cookies, it's easier to remove the excess than to shift them onto the baking sheets once they are rolled and cut with a cutter. Artists use the term relief sculpture to describe this procedure. What you're doing is removing what doesn't belong in order to make room for what does. All you have to do is invert the cookie sheet after rolling and cutting the cookies on waxed paper.

Thumbprints and biscotti are traditional varieties of cookies that are included in this chapter in addition to rolled-dough cookies. While they don't require a rolling pin-like piece of equipment, they are shaped by hand to provide a consistent appearance.

Note: Unless otherwise stated, follow the following storage instructions for cookies: At room temperature, store cookies in an airtight container with waxed paper or parchment sheets between them.

days. For up to two months, cookies that haven't been frosted can be thrown away.

Cookies with Sugar for the Holidays

Cookies like this are to Christmas what a blank canvas is to a painter.

There are countless options available to you from this point on. Sugar cookies are rich in buttery flavor and crisp when they're first taken out of the oven.

Depending on the size of the cutters used, this recipe will yield 2 to 4 dozen. 30 minutes of active time

38   CHRISTMAS BASED GLUTEN-FREE RECIPES

13/4 hours from start to end, including 1 hour for dough cooling Amaranth flour, 1 and a half cups

Confectioners' sugar is 1 cup.

cornstarch, half a cup

xanthan gum, 1 teaspoon

1-teaspoon tartaric acid

Salt is a good addition.

2 sticks unsalted butter, thinly sliced, about half a pound a single, big egg

Whole milk in a spoonful

1 tsp. of pure vanilla essence

A sweet rice flour

icing sugar and water (optional)

Icing made with buttercream (optional) Candy decorations that are free of gluten (optional)

1. In a food processor fitted with a steel blade, combine amaranth flour, confectioners' sugar, cornstarch, xanthan gum, cream of tartar, and salt. Blend for about 5 seconds, then remove the blades. Then, using an on-and-off pulsing motion, pulse the butter into the mixture until it resembles coarse grain.

ICING 39

In a small cup, whisk together the egg, milk, and vanilla extract. Drizzle a liquid into the food.

10 times in a food processor until a stiff dough forms in the mixing dish Add additional milk in 1-teaspoon increments if the dough is dry and doesn't form a ball.

The dough should be divided in half and wrapped in plastic wrap. Make a pancake out of the dough by flattening it out with your hands. It's best to keep it in the fridge for an hour or so to firm up (or up to 2 days).

The oven should be preheated to 350°F. Using parchment paper or silicone baking mats, cover two baking sheets with the mixture.

Apply a light dusting of sweet rice flour to waxed paper, as well as a rolling pin. Roll out the dough to a 1/4-inch thickness. Dip cookie cutters in sweet rice flour, and cut out cookies with them. Transfer the cookies to the baking pans after removing any extra dough. Re-roll any leftover dough, and chill it for an additional 15 minutes if needed.

6. Bake the cookies for about 10 to 12 minutes, or until the edges are brown. Cool cookies for 2 people

cooling racks after they've been sitting on the baking sheets for at least five minutes before they can be moved. Decorate cooled cookies with royal icing and candies, if you choose.

40 CHRISTMAS BASED GLUTEN-FREE RECIPES

Variations

Lemon oil can be substituted for vanilla essence and 2 teaspoons of grated lemon zest can be added to the bread dough.

Alternate half of the amaranth flour with 1/2 cup almond meal and use almond extract instead of vanilla essence in this recipe.

It can be challenging to handle gluten-free dough since it softens more quickly than dough made with wheat flour. The sheets of rolled-out dough can be put in the freezer for 10 to 15 minutes to stiffen them up a bit.

Chapter Five

GINGERBREAD LITTLE HUMANS

These traditional cookies can be painted before baking or adorned after baking with a variety of delicious spices.

Approximately 2 to 3 dozen servings, depending on the size of the cutters used. 30 minutes of active time

13/4 hours from start to end, including 1 hour for dough cooling 1 pound of brown rice

Cornstarch is 1 cup in volume.

Ground ginger: 2 tablespoons

Nutmeg, freshly grated, to taste

1/8 tsp. cinnamon powder

Zanthan gum is 1/2 teaspoon.

Half a teaspoon of baking powder.

Salt with a quarter teaspoon

42 CHRISTMAS BASED GLUTEN-FREE RECIPES

Unsalted butter, softened to 6 tablespoons (3/4 stick) 1/3 of a cup of granulated sugar

Dark molasses in half a cup

Vanilla extract in its purest form:

A sweet rice flour

Icing with a royal touch

Candies that are devoid of gluten (optional)

Baking soda and salt should be added to the rice flour mixture together with the other dry ingredients. Make a thorough stir.

Using an electric mixer on low speed, whip the butter and confectioners' sugar together in a second bowl. Beat for three to four beats at a fast speed.

till frothy and light, about a minute or two Beat the molasses and vanilla in for a minute before serving.

As you begin to incorporate the dry ingredients into the butter mixture, beat until a stiff dough forms.

Wrap each half of the dough in plastic and refrigerate. Make a pancake out of the dough by flattening it out with your hands.

Serve immediately or store in the refrigerator for up to 2 days.

The oven should be preheated to 350°F. Using parchment paper or silicone baking mats, cover two baking sheets with the mixture.

GINGERBREAD LITTLE HUMANS

Apply a light dusting of sweet rice flour to waxed paper, as well as a rolling pin. Roll out the dough to a 1/4-inch thickness. Dip cookie cutters in sweet rice flour, and cut out cookies with them. Transfer the cookies to the baking pans after removing any extra dough. Re-roll any leftover dough, and chill it for an additional 15 minutes if needed.

In a baking sheet, combine the cookie ingredients and bake for 10-12 minutes, or until set. Cool cookies on the baking sheets for 2 minutes, then transfer them to cooling racks with a spatula to finish cooling. Decorate the cooled cookies with royal icing and candies.

Variation

Bake the cookies as drop cookies for 13 to 15 minutes, with 1/2 cup chopped raisins added to the mixture. Drop cookies don't need to be chilled.

Chapter Six

SPRITZ

Nordic baking is the inspiration behind Spritz. Cookie presses are used to create these wacky forms out of cookie dough. Almond flavoring and almond meal are used in the dough for this variation of the cookie.

About three to four dozen.

20 minutes of active time

One-and-a-half hours from start to finish, including an hour to chill the dough 1 cup rice flour, white

Confectioners' sugar is 1 cup.

2 tablespoons of brown sugar

a half-cup of potato flour

Almond meal in half a cup

xanthan gum, 1 teaspoon

Salt with a quarter teaspoon

46 CHRISTMAS BASED GLUTEN-FREE RECIPES

Sliced 1/2 pound of unsalted butter (equivalent to two sticks)

a single, big egg

Egg whites, about 1 pound

1 tsp. of pure vanilla essence

Pure almond extract in a half teaspoon

Sugar sprinkles that are free of gluten

Candies that are devoid of gluten.

cherries coated in icing

In a food processor fitted with a steel blade, combine white rice flour, confectioners' sugar, sweet rice flour, potato starch, almond meal, xanthan gum, and salt.

Blend for about 5 seconds, then remove the blades. Then, using an on-and-off pulsing motion, pulse the butter into the mixture until it resembles coarse grain.

In a small cup, mix together the egg, egg white, vanilla, and almond extract. About 10 times, or until a stiff dough forms, drizzle in the liquid. If the dough is too dry to form a ball, add a small amount of milk at a time, starting with a teaspoon at a time.

Wrap each half of the dough with plastic wrap. Make a pancake out of the dough by flattening it out with your hands. For up to two days, refrigerate the dough.

The oven should be preheated to 350°F. Using parchment paper or silicone baking mats, cover two baking sheets with the mixture.

5. Use a cookie press to transfer the dough to the baking sheets. You can decorate with a variety of sweets, including sugar sprinkles, candies, and candied cherries.

6. Bake the cookies for about 10 to 12 minutes, or until the edges are brown. Cool cookies for 2 people

cooling racks after they've been sitting on the baking sheets for at least five minutes before they can be moved.

Variations

In place of vanilla and almond extracts, use 1 tablespoon of grated lemon zest and 1 tablespoon of lemon oil in the dough

Replace almond flour with hazelnut flour.

Even if you don't own a cookie press, you can still create beautiful and unique cookies. When using a basic tip, make wreath-shaped circles out of the dough using a pastry bag fitted with a star tip. Afterwards, decorate and bake!

Chapter Seven

LINZER COOKIES

Cookies made by the Austrian company Linzer

A cutout in the cookie's top allows you to glimpse the luscious raspberry jam that holds the layers together.

Amount Produced: Two dozen

30 minutes of active time

13/4 hours from start to end, including 1 hour for dough cooling 1 12 cups of white rice powder

34 cup ground almonds

Xanthan gum in 11/4 tsp.

3/4 tsp. baking powder without gluten

12 tsp. of salt

Softened unsalted butter, 1/4 pound (1 stick)

3/4 cup of sugar, granulated

50 CHRISTMAS BASED GLUTEN-FREE RECIPES

a single, big egg

Whole milk in a spoonful

almond extract, about 34 of a teaspoon

A sweet rice flour

The seedless raspberry jam is 3/4 cup.

1/3 of a cup of granulated sugar

The first step is to mix together the rice flour, almond meal, xanthan gum, baking powder, and salt in a large basin. Make a thorough stir.

Using an electric mixer, whip the butter and sugar together in a second bowl. Beat at high speed for 3 to 4 minutes, or until the mixture is light and fluffier. Beat for a minute after adding the egg, milk, and almond extract.

As you begin to incorporate the dry ingredients into the butter mixture, beat until a stiff dough forms.

Put the dough in a plastic bag. Make a pancake out of the dough by flattening it out with your hands. For up to two days, refrigerate the dough.

The oven should be preheated to 350°F. Using parchment paper or silicone baking mats, cover two baking sheets with the mixture.

LINZER COOKIES   51

Apply a light dusting of sweet rice flour to waxed paper, as well as a rolling pin. 1/8-inch-thick dough should be rolled out. Cut out 48 cookies using a 2-inch flower-shaped cookie cutter dipped in sweet rice flour. Transfer the cookies to the baking pans after removing any extra dough. Cut out 24 cookies using a 3/4-inch cutter. Re-roll any leftover dough, and chill it for an additional 15 minutes if needed.

In order to brown the edges, bake the cookies for 8 to 10 minutes. Cool cookies for 2 people

cooling racks after they've been sitting on the baking sheets for at least five minutes before they can be moved.

7. Apply jam to the 24 cookies without holes by sprinkling them with it. Apply confectioner's sugar to the remaining cookies. Top the jam-covered cookies with cookies with holes.

Variation

Rather than using jam, use melted white or dark chocolate instead.

Cookie variations of Austria's most well-known sweet treat, Linzertorte. Written recipes for this dish date back to the early eighteenth century and are said to have originated in the Austrian city of Linz. In Austria, the pastry is filled with black currant preserves, although in North America, the filling is frequently raspberry.

52 CHRISTMAS BASED GLUTEN-FREE RECIPES

Ornaments made with lemon sugar cookies

Crispy cookies with a citrus flavor are part of a popular cookie trend called as

"Cookies from the refrigerator." Because the dough is chilled in a log form and baked in rounds, it's simple to scale up production.

A total of three dozen can be made from this recipe.

20 minutes of active time

One-and-a-half hours from start to finish, including an hour to chill the dough 1 12 cups of white rice powder

1.5 cups powdered sugar

cornstarch, 1/3 cup

Tapioca starch, one-third of a cup

1-teaspoon tartaric acid

Baking soda

Xanthan gum in a quarter teaspoon

Salt with a quarter teaspoon

Sliced unsalted butter, about half a pound (2 sticks) a single, big egg

Whole milk in a spoonful

Grate 2 teaspoons of lemon zest into the mixture.

Lemon oil in a half teaspoon

Candies and sugar sprinkles free of gluten (optional) In a food processor fitted with a steel blade, combine rice flour, confectioners' sugar, cornstarch, tapioca starch, cream of tartar, baking soda, xanthan gum, and salt.

Blend for about 5 seconds, then remove the blades. Then, using an on-and-off pulsing motion, pulse the butter into the mixture until it resembles coarse grain.

2. In a small cup, whisk together the egg, milk, lemon zest, and lemon oil.

About 10 times, or until a stiff dough forms, drizzle in the liquid.

If the dough is too dry and won't come together, add 1 teaspoon of milk at a time until it does.

Form the dough into a 21/2-inch-diameter log on a waxed paper sheet. For up to 2 hours, refrigerate the dough covered in plastic wrap.

days.

The oven should be preheated to 350°F. Using parchment paper or silicone baking mats, cover two baking sheets with the mixture.

54 CHRISTMAS BASED GLUTEN-FREE RECIPES

Using a serrated knife, slice the cold dough into 1/4-inch pieces and place them on the baking sheets. Sugar crystals can be used to decorate cookies, if desired.

6. Bake the cookies for about 10 to 12 minutes, or until the edges are brown. Cool cookies for 2 people

cooling racks after they've been sitting on the baking sheets for at least five minutes before they can be moved.

Variation

Make a substitution for the lemon oil and lemon zest with lime oil.

These cookies can be hung from a tiny tree. Using a paring knife, make a small hole at the top of the cookie and check to see if the holes have closed up after baking. After the cookies have cooled, thread a ribbon through the hole.

Spiced Peppermint Spindles

Combining pink dough scented with peppermint and white dough creates a delightful cookie that looks tougher to prepare than it is.

Peppermint is a staple of the holiday season, and now you can enjoy it in a new way.

Amount Produced: Two dozen

20 minutes of active time

LINZER COOKIES 55

33/4 hours from start to finish, including 3 hours for the dough to cool. White rice flour, 11.5 ounces

1/2 a cup of granulated sugar

Potato starch is 1/4 cup.

xanthan gum, 1 teaspoon

Half a teaspoon of baking powder.

Salt with a quarter teaspoon

1 large egg, thinly sliced with 1/4 pound (1 stick) unsalted butter

The yolk of a single egg

1/2 tsp. oil of peppermint or pure extract of peppermint 3 to 5 drops of red food dye.

In a food processor fitted with a steel blade, combine rice flour, confectioners' sugar, potato starch, xanthan gum, baking soda, and salt. Blend for about 5 seconds, then remove the blades. Then, using an on-and-off pulsing motion, pulse the butter into the mixture until it resembles coarse grain.

In a small cup, mix together the egg and the egg yolk. About 10 times, or until a stiff dough forms, drizzle in the liquid.

In step three, take out half of the dough from the food processor and put it aside. Process the dough until it is a

56 CHRISTMAS BASED GLUTEN-FREE RECIPES

uniform shade of green after adding the peppermint oil and food coloring to the food processor.

Each dough disc should be individually wrapped in plastic wrap to prevent leaking. Make a pancake out of the dough by flattening it out with your hands. Allow the dough to rest for one hour in the refrigerator.

It can be kept in the fridge for up to two days.

4. Separately roll out each piece of dough to a thickness of about 1/4 inch. Put the white dough on top of the peppermint dough and press the two together around the perimeter.

Roll the dough into a log using a piece of waxed paper or a flexible cutting board as a guide. Refrigerate for two hours after wrapping in plastic wrap.

The oven should be preheated to 350°F. Using parchment paper or silicone baking mats, cover two baking sheets with the mixture.

Six. Slice the cold dough into 1/4-inch-thick slices with a serrated knife and place them on the baking sheets.

7. Bake cookies for 10 to 12 minutes or until sides are golden. Cool cookies for 2 people

cooling racks after they've been sitting on the baking sheets for at least five minutes before they can be moved.

Variation

LINZER COOKIES   57

Add 1/2 cup crushed peppermint candies to the vanilla dough and substitute green food coloring for the red food coloring.

Plastic wrap is a must for refrigerating the log for the second time around. The dough may dry out and be difficult to cut if it isn't held in place properly.

Chapter Eight

GINGERBREAD FINGERS

Shortbread is a British tradition, and these spritely candied ginger-flavored bites are thick and crispy, with a surprising texture.

Amount Produced: Two dozen

At least 25 minutes of active time

13/4 hours from start to end, including 1 hour for dough cooling Brown rice flour is 2 cups.

Sweet rice flour is 1/3 of a cup.

a third of a cup of almond flour

xanthan gum, 1 teaspoon

12 tsp. of salt

a half pound (2 sticks) of softened unsalted butter

1/3 cup dark brown sugar that has been tightly packed

Finely sliced crystallized ginger in half a cup

60   CHRISTMAS BASED GLUTEN-FREE RECIPES

Vanilla extract in its purest form:

A sweet rice flour

When you're ready to bake, combine all of the dry ingredients except the xanthan gum and salt in a large basin. Make a thorough stir.

Using an electric mixer, whip the butter and sugar together in a second bowl. Beat at high speed for 3 to 4 minutes, or until the mixture is light and fluffier. Beat in the vanilla and crystallized ginger for a minute.

Once you've got a firm dough, slowly put in the dry ingredients. Put the dough in a plastic bag. Make a pancake out of the dough by flattening it out with your hands. For up to two days, refrigerate the dough.

The oven should be preheated to 350°F. Using parchment paper or silicone baking mats, cover two baking sheets with the mixture.

Apply a light dusting of sweet rice flour to waxed paper, as well as a rolling pin. Roll out the dough to a half-inch thickness. Cut into 4-inch by 1-inch rectangles.

Bake the cookies on the baking pans as instructed. Re-roll any leftover dough, and chill it for an additional 15 minutes if needed.

GINGERBREAD FINGERS   61

The edges of the cookies should be golden brown after 12 to 15 minutes of baking. Cool cookies for 2 people

cooling racks after they've been sitting on the baking sheets for at least five minutes before they can be moved.

Variations

Adding dried currants or apricots to the dough is simple.

Using white chocolate and colored sugars, dip one end of cooled cookies.

Fresh ginger is candied in sugar syrup to preserve it as crystallized ginger. Coarse sugar is then added to the mixture. If you can't find it in the spice section, you can usually find it in bulk at most health food stores.

Chapter Nine

NUTELLA COOKIES

Nutella and peanut butter thumbprints in chocolate

Cookies

It's never too late to bring back old favorites for the holidays if you dress them up a bit. This cookie is no exception. A chocolate candy is placed on top of the peanut butter dough.

Amount Produced: Two dozen

20 minutes of active time

45 minutes from start to finish

Flour made from the amaranth plant

Potato starch is 1/4 cup.

Zanthan gum is 1/2 teaspoon.

Half a teaspoon of baking powder.

Salt is a good addition.

64 CHRISTMAS BASED GLUTEN-FREE RECIPES

a half stick of softened unsalted butter Light brown sugar, 3/4 cup, tightly packed

Peanut butter, half a cup, smooth

a single, big egg

Vanilla extract in its purest form:

Unwrapped chocolate kisses, 24 count

The oven should be preheated to 350°F. Using parchment paper or silicone baking mats, cover two baking sheets with the mixture.

Gather the ingredients for the amaranth flour, potato starch, xanthan gum, baking soda and salt in a bowl and combine thoroughly. Make a thorough stir.

Beat the butter and sugar together on low speed in a separate mixing bowl until well combined. Beat at high speed for 3 to 4 minutes, or until the mixture is light and fluffier. Beat in the egg, peanut butter, and vanilla for a minute.

To make stiff dough, add dry ingredients one at a time while continuing to beat the butter mixture.

Then, using your hands, form the dough into small balls and place them on the prepared baking sheets. If the dough is too soft to roll, place it in the refrigerator for a few minutes. Place a candy in the center of each ball after making an indentation with the tip of your finger.

NUTELLA COOKIES 65

To ensure that the cookies are firm to the touch, bake for 12-14 minutes. Cool cookies for 2 people

cooling racks after they've been sitting on the baking sheets for at least five minutes before they can be moved.

Variations

Instead of peanut butter, use sweetened almond butter, pure almond extract instead of vanilla, and 1/2 cup almond meal in place of 1/2 cup amaranth flour.

Replace the candies in the center of the cookies with 3/4 teaspoon of fruit jelly.

Chapter Ten

CANDIED CHERRY AND WALNUTS

Thumbprints in Candied Cherry and Walnut

Cookies

Cookie lovers of all ages adore these confections because of their crunchy nut coating and eye-catching cherry garnish.

A total of three dozen can be made from this recipe.

20 minutes of active time

Fifty minutes from beginning to end:

1 12 cups of white rice powder

Confectioners' sugar is 1 cup.

cornstarch, half a cup

xanthan gum, 1 teaspoon

1-teaspoon tartaric acid

Salt is a good addition.

68 CHRISTMAS BASED GLUTEN-FREE RECIPES

2 sticks unsalted butter, thinly sliced, about half a pound a single, big egg

Whole milk in a spoonful

1 tsp. of pure vanilla essence

Finely chopped walnuts make up one cup of the ingredient.

Sixteen half-pints of red or green candied cherries

The oven should be preheated to 350°F. Using parchment paper or silicone baking mats, cover two baking sheets with the mixture.

A food processor fitted with a steel blade can be used to combine rice flour, confectioner's sugar, cornstarch, xanthan gum, cream of tartar, and salt. Blend for about 5 seconds, then remove the blades. Then, using an on-and-off pulsing motion, pulse the butter into the mixture until it resembles coarse grain.

Whisk the egg, milk, and vanilla together in a small cup. About 10 times, or until a stiff dough forms, drizzle in the liquid. Add additional milk in 1-teaspoon increments if the dough is dry and doesn't form a ball.

Make a waxed paper sheet by putting walnuts on it. Roll out the dough into balls, coat them in walnuts, and place them on the baking sheets. If the dough is too soft to roll, place it in the

CANDIED CHERRY AND WALNUTS

refrigerator for a few minutes. Place 1 in the center of each ball after making an indentation with your fingertip.

Domed side up, place the cherry in the depression.

5) Bake the cookies for 12 to 14 minutes, or until they are firm to the touch. Cool cookies for 2 people

cooling racks after they've been sitting on the baking sheets for at least five minutes before they can be moved.

Variation

Half a teaspoon of strawberry or raspberry jam can be used in place of the cherry portion.

Cream of tartar is made from the acid that accumulates in wine barrels over time. Baking soda is combined with it to create the same chemical reaction as baking powder.

Chapter Eleven

BISCOTTI WITH ALMONDS

The almonds, almond meal in the dough, and aromatic almond extract all contribute to the almond flavor of these treats.

Amount Produced: Two dozen

20 minutes of active time

Thirteen and a half hours.

1.5 cups almonds, sliced

Brown rice flour is half a cup.

Almond meal in half a cup

Potato starch is a third of a cup

1 cup tapioca starch 3 tblsp

xanthan gum, 1 teaspoon

1/2 tsp. baking powder without gluten

72 CHRISTMAS BASED GLUTEN-FREE RECIPES

Salt with a quarter teaspoon

Softened unsalted butter, 1/4 pound (1 stick)

Confectioner's sugar: 11/4 cups

Eggs of a large size

The pure almond extract is 1 teaspoon in volume.

The oven should be preheated to 350°F. Line a baking sheet with parchment paper or a silicone baking mat and then bake as directed.

5. To toast almonds, place them on a baking pan for 5 to 7 minutes, or until they begin to brown. Set aside the nuts after they've finished roasting.

Then, in a large bowl, whisk together the rice flour, xanthan gum, tapioca starch, xanthan gum, baking powder, and salt. Make a thorough stir.

With an electric mixer on low speed, mix together the butter and confectioners' sugar in another bowl. Beat for three to four beats at a fast speed.

till frothy and light, about a minute or two One minute later, add the eggs and almond essence, and mix thoroughly.

To produce a dough, gradually add flour to butter mixture and beat until it becomes stiff.

The dough will be better if the almonds are folded in.

BISCOTTI WITH ALMONDS   73

6. Shape the dough into a 12-inch-long, 3-inch-wide log and place it on the baking sheet that has been prepared. A light golden color should be achieved in around 40 minutes of baking time. Allow to cool for a minimum of 30 minutes before using.

The log should be placed on a cutting board. Use a sharp, serrated knife to slice the log into 1/2- to 3/4-inch-thick slices on the diagonal. On a baking sheet, arrange biscotti so that the sliced side is facing up.

Bake for 15 minutes, or until the tops are just beginning to turn a soft golden color. Cool the biscotti on a cooling rack before serving.

Don't bake the biscotti a second time if you prefer a softer texture.

Allow the log to cool for five minutes before chopping it.

Italians eat these biscotti all year round, not just during the Christmas season.

Biscotti flavored with chocolate and peppermint.

The classic Christmas flavor combination of chocolate and peppermint is brought to life in this biscotti recipe, which is topped with frosting and crushed candy canes to amp up the minty freshness.

Amount Produced: Two dozen

74 CHRISTMAS BASED GLUTEN-FREE RECIPES

At least 25 minutes of active time

2 hours from beginning to end.

1 pound of brown rice

1/2 cup chocolate powder, unsweetened

Potato starch is a third of a cup

1 cup tapioca starch 3 tblsp

xanthan gum, 1 teaspoon

1/2 tsp. baking powder without gluten

Salt with a quarter teaspoon

Softened unsalted butter, 1/4 pound (1 stick)

2 and a half cups of granulated sugar split

Eggs of a large size

1 (3-ounce) container softened cream cheese, 1/8 teaspoon pure peppermint oil or extract

a half cup of chopped peppermint candies

The oven should be preheated to 350°F. Line a baking sheet with parchment paper or a silicone baking mat and then bake as directed.

Baking powder and salt are added to a bowl along with the rice flour and cocoa powder. Make a thorough stir.

BISCOTTI WITH ALMONDS 75

With an electric mixer on low speed, combine the butter and 11/4 cups of confectioners' sugar in a separate bowl. Beat for three to four beats at a fast speed.

till frothy and light, about a minute or two Beat for a minute after adding the eggs and half a teaspoon of peppermint oil.

To make stiff dough, add dry ingredients one at a time while continuing to beat the butter mixture.

5. Shape the dough into a 12-inch-long, 3-inch-wide log and place it on the baking sheet that has been prepared. A light golden color should be achieved in around 40 minutes of baking time. Allow to cool for a minimum of 30 minutes before using.

A cutting board should be placed on top of the log in order to cut it. Use a sharp, serrated knife to slice the log into 1/2- to 3/4-inch-thick slices on the diagonal. On a baking sheet, arrange biscotti so that the sliced side is facing up.

Bake for 15 minutes, or until the tops are just beginning to turn a soft golden color. Cool the biscotti on a cooling rack before serving.

For the frosting, put the cream cheese, the remaining sugar, and the remaining peppermint oil in a dish and whisk until smooth. A low-speed electric mixer can be used to blend the ingredients. Beat on high for 2 to 3 minutes, or until fluffy and light in color.

76   CHRISTMAS BASED GLUTEN-FREE RECIPES

Frost thin edges of cookies, then add crushed peppermint candies to the icing.

Variation

Replace the peppermint extract with vanilla extract, add 1 tablespoon of instant espresso powder to the dough, and omit the crushed peppermint candies in favor of micro chocolate chips.

Chapter Twelve

PISTACHIO BISCOTTI

Biscotti for the season of goodwill

These crisp cookies are decorated with pistachio nuts and dried cranberries in festive green and red.

Amount Produced: Two dozen

20 minutes of active time

Thirteen and a half hours.

1 pound of brown rice

Potato starch is a third of a cup

1 cup tapioca starch 3 tblsp

xanthan gum, 1 teaspoon

1/2 tsp. baking powder without gluten

Salt with a quarter teaspoon

Softened unsalted butter, 1/4 pound (1 stick)

78 CHRISTMAS BASED GLUTEN-FREE RECIPES

Confectioner's sugar: 11/4 cups

Eggs of a large size

1 tsp. of pure vanilla essence

Pistachios cut into 3/4 cup.

1 cup cranberries, drained and dried

The oven should be preheated to 350°F. Line a baking sheet with parchment paper or a silicone baking mat and then bake as directed.

A mixing bowl should be used to mix together rice flour, potato starch, tapioca starch, baking powder and salt. Make a thorough stir.

With an electric mixer, cream the butter and confectioners' sugar together in a separate basin until smooth. Beat for three to four beats at a fast speed.

till frothy and light, about a minute or two One minute after putting in eggs and vanilla extract, whisk the mixture.

To make stiff dough, add dry ingredients one at a time while continuing to beat the butter mixture.

The dough should include pistachios and cranberries.

5. Shape the dough into a 12-inch-long, 3-inch-wide log and place it on the baking sheet that has been prepared. A light golden color should be achieved in around 40 minutes of

baking time. Allow to cool for a minimum of 30 minutes before using.

A cutting board should be placed on top of the log in order to cut it. Use a sharp, serrated knife to slice the log into 1/2- to 3/4-inch-thick slices on the diagonal. On a baking sheet, arrange biscotti so that the sliced side is facing up.

Bake for 15 minutes, or until the tops are just beginning to turn a soft golden color. Cool the biscotti on a cooling rack before serving.

In the absence of cooling racks, bake the cookies first on the rack, then move them to plastic wrap dusted with granulated sugar. The sugar will help protect the bottoms from becoming stuck.

There is nothing about drop cookies that screams "Christmas cookie" by themselves.

Due to their unusual shape, they are rarely decorated with colorful frosting, although they can be adorned with small candies. However, this category includes some of our favorite cookies, such as chocolate chip and oatmeal raisin. You'll find a variety of hearty dishes in this chapter, such as these.

After the dough has been produced, children have traditionally been given the duty of portioning out the cookie dough. Drop cookies, on the other hand, necessitate regular mounds in order to be a success. The circumference and

80 CHRISTMAS BASED GLUTEN-FREE RECIPES

height of a circle are both considered when determining its size.

Bake time is the only difference between chewy and crisp cookies if cookies are of equal size. There are a few minutes in each of these recipes. You'll get a moister and chewier cookie if you bake them for a shorter period of time rather than letting them bake for the entire length of time, which will cause most of the moisture to evaporate.

As a verb, "drop" is a little misleading in some cases. While the dough is softer than for rolled cookies, it actually doesn't drop onto the baking sheets without some coaxing. Either another spoon or a finger will do the trick here. Spray both spoons with vegetable oil spray before employing the "two-spoon approach" to make it easier to remove the dough. The following is a list of other tips for baking drop cookies:

Running the back of your cookie sheets under cold water after each batch can help keep them cool. Cookies flatten when placed on a warm baking pan after being made in the traditional manner.

• Make a mental note of the distance between the cookie dough mounds as you arrange them on the baking sheet. There are some cookies that spread a lot more than others.

If you're using cookie sheets, rotate them halfway through the baking time to ensure even baking. •

PISTACHIO BISCOTTI   81

sheets of paper Cookies baked on the upper rack brown more quickly than those baked on the bottom rack, even when using a convection fan.

• Before moving cookies to cooling racks, always allow them to cool for two minutes on the baking sheets.

Note: Unless otherwise stated, follow the following storage instructions for cookies: At room temperature, store cookies in an airtight container with waxed paper or parchment sheets between them.

days. If not decorated, cookies can be stored in the freezer for up to two months.

Chapter Thirteen

CAKE ICING

Mexican Wedding Cookies is another name for these. They have a crispy, buttery exterior and are adorned with confectioners' sugar.

A total of three dozen can be made from this recipe.

15 minutes of active time

30 minutes from start to finish

Chopped pecans, about 1 cup

1 12 cups of white rice powder

Potato starch is 1/4 cup.

one and a quarter cups of sweetened rice flour

Zanthan gum is 1/2 teaspoon.

12 tsp. of salt

Unsalted butter in the amount of 1/2 pound

84 CHRISTMAS BASED GLUTEN-FREE RECIPES

1 and a half cups granulated sugar, divided

1 tsp. of pure vanilla essence

The oven should be preheated to 350°F. Using parchment paper or silicone baking mats, cover two baking sheets with the mixture. Toast pecans on a baking sheet for 5 to 7 minutes, or until they begin to brown. Set aside for now. The oven temperature should be lowered to 325°F.

In a mixing bowl, combine the rice flour, potato starch, sweet rice flour, xanthan gum, and salt. Make a thorough stir.

Using an electric mixer on low speed, whip the butter and 1 cup of confectioners' sugar together in a second bowl. Beat at high speed for 3 to 4 minutes, or until the mixture is light and fluffier. For one minute, beat in the vanilla extract.

To make stiff dough, add dry ingredients one at a time while continuing to beat the butter mixture.

Then, add the pecans.

Form 1-tablespoon mounds of dough onto the baking sheets, about 1 1/2 inches apart. Bake for about 15 minutes. Bake cookies for about 15 to 20 minutes, or until they're just beginning to brown on the outside. Set aside the pan for 2 minutes to cool.

In a shallow basin, combine the remaining 1/2 cup of confectioners' sugar. Cool cookies entirely on a cooling rack after being dusted with confectioners' sugar.

Variations

Sweetened coconut can be used in place of pecans.

Replace the vanilla with 1 tablespoon of grated orange zest.

Pure vanilla extract must contain one pound of vanilla beans per gallon in order to meet FDA guidelines, which explains why it is twice as expensive as fake extract. Given how little you use, it's certainly a good investment. Before you buy anything, be sure you read the labels.

Chapter Fourteen

BRAZILIAN SWEETS

Brazilian cornstarch brand Biscoitos de Maizena is the inspiration for these cookies, which in Portuguese are known as Biscoitos de Maizena. You can whip up a batch in a matter of minutes and they'll practically melt in your mouth.

A total of three dozen can be made from this recipe.

15 minutes of active time

30 minutes from start to finish

Cornstarch is 2 1/2 cups.

3/4 cup finely chopped brown sugar

12 tsp. of salt

Sliced unsalted butter, about half a pound (2 sticks) a single, big egg

1 big yolk of an egg

Vanilla extract in the amount of 3/4 teaspoon

88   CHRISTMAS BASED GLUTEN-FREE RECIPES

The oven should be preheated to 375°F. Using parchment paper or silicone baking mats, cover two baking sheets with the mixture.

2. In a food processor fitted with a steel blade, combine cornstarch, sugar, and salt.

Blend for about 5 seconds, then remove the blades. Then, using an on-and-off pulsing motion, pulse the butter into the mixture until it resembles coarse grain.

In a small cup, mix together the egg, the egg yolk, and the vanilla extract. About 10 times, or until a stiff dough forms, drizzle in the liquid. If the dough is too dry to form a ball, add a small amount of milk at a time, starting with a teaspoon at a time.

Transfer 1-tablespoon-sized balls of dough to the baking sheets, allowing at least 2 inches between each ball. Fork tines can be used to flatten balls into a crosshatch pattern.

Take it out and let it cool for a few minutes before moving on to step 5. Cookies can be cooled on baking sheets.

Transfer to a wire rack to cool entirely after cooling for two minutes.

Variation

Instead of vanilla, use pure almond extract, and use 1/2 cup almond meal instead of 1/2 cup cornstarch.

It was patented in the United States in 1841 by Orlando Jones, a Scotsman who had been selling cornstarch since 1840 in Paisley, Scotland. Brown & Polson Corn Flour was fixed at 5 pence every 1/4-pound container in Ireland during the "Emergency," as the Irish called World War II.

Dried Fruit Cornbread

Cookies prepared with cornmeal and rum-soaked dried fruit are truly out of the ordinary. For Thanksgiving and Christmas, these are a great option.

A total of three dozen can be made from this recipe.

15 minutes of active time

40 minutes from start to finish

Golden raisins in a quarter-cup measure

Dried cranberries in 1/4 cup

a quarter-cup of cherry preserves

1/4 cup of rum

Cornmeal is 1 1/2 cups.

One and a half cup of cornstarch

3/4 cup of sugar, granulated

1 tsp. baking powder without gluten

Zanthan gum is 1/2 teaspoon.

CHRISTMAS BASED GLUTEN-FREE RECIPES

12 tsp. of salt

Sliced unsalted butter, 1/4 pound

Eggs of a large size

2 tbsp. full-fat dairy milk

1 tablespoon of finely shredded orange peel

Vanilla extract in its purest form:

The oven should be preheated to 350°F. Using parchment paper or silicone baking mats, cover two baking sheets with the mixture. Toss the rum-coated golden raisins, dried cranberries, and dried cherries in a small mixing dish.

Second, put the steel blade in a food processor with the ingredients for the cornmeal and cornstarch. Blend for about 5 seconds, then remove the blades. Then, using an on-and-off pulsing motion, pulse the butter into the mixture until it resembles coarse grain.

In a small cup, whisk together the eggs, milk, orange zest, and vanilla extract.

About 10 times, or until a stiff dough forms, drizzle in the liquid.

Add additional milk in 1-teaspoon increments if the dough is dry and doesn't form a ball.

4. Add fruit and any remaining rum to the bowl after scraping the dough into it.

5. Place the dough on the prepared baking sheets, 1 spoonful at a time, 2 inches apart from one another. A cookie should be dry after baking for 20 to 25 minutes. Cool cookies for 2 people

Then transfer to a wire rack and allow to cool completely before serving.

Variations

Some of the dried fruits can be replaced by toasting 1/3 cup chopped walnuts at 350°F for 5 to 7 minutes.

Dried fruits can be replaced with chopped candied citrus peels and candied cherries.

When you need to grate a lot of citrus zest, you can save time by using a vegetable peeler to separate the colored zest from the white pith beneath it. Using a mini-food processor, mince the strips into a fine paste.

Chapter Fifteen

PEANUT BUTTER COOKIES

Brown sugar adds a distinct depth of flavor to this gluten-free rendition of a beloved family recipe.

Produces two to three dozen

20 minutes of active time

35 minutes from the start until the end

1 pound of brown rice

Tapioca flour is 1/4 cup.

Cornstarch is 1/4 cup.

11/4 tsp. baking powder without gluten

Zanthan gum is 1/2 teaspoon.

12 tsp. of salt

Softened unsalted butter, 1/4 pound (1 stick)

1 jar of creamy PB (either smooth or chunky)

94 CHRISTMAS BASED GLUTEN-FREE RECIPES

Sugar in the form of granular

1/2 cup dark brown sugar, tightly packed

a single, big egg

1 big yolk of an egg

Vanilla extract in its purest form:

The oven should be preheated to 375°F. Using parchment paper or silicone baking mats, cover two baking sheets with the mixture.

Pour the following ingredients into a mixing bowl: rice flour, tapioca flour, xanthan gum, baking powder, and salt. Make a thorough stir.

A third mixing bowl should be used to whip up the mixture of peanut butter, granulated sugar and brown sugar, using an electric mixer on low speed. Beat at high speed for 3 to 4 minutes, or until the mixture is light and fluffier. Add the egg, the yolk, then the white.

Vanilla and beat for one minute.

To make stiff dough, add dry ingredients one at a time while continuing to beat the butter mixture.

To bake, divide the dough into 1-tablespoon portions and roll into balls. Place on prepared baking sheets, spacing them apart by 2 inches. Fork tines can be used to flatten balls into a crosshatch pattern.

It should be done in 8 to 10 minutes. Allow cookies to cool for two minutes on the baking sheets before transferring to a wire rack to finish cooling.

Variations

Before baking, mix in 1 cup of chocolate chips to the batter.

Replace peanut butter with almond or cashew butter.

To replace the region's cotton crop, which had been devastated by the boll weevil, Tuskegee Institute lecturer George Washington Carver advocated for the use of peanuts. In the year 1916,

The Peanut: Its Growing and Preparation in 105 Recipes, a Scientific Research Bulletin

He provided three recipes for peanut cookies that called for crushed or chopped peanuts as an ingredient in the book for Human Consumption. The first time that peanut butter was specified as an ingredient in cookies was in the early 1920s.

Chapter Sixteen

PINA COLADA OATMEAL COOKIES

As a cookie and as a drink, the combination of pineapple, coconut, and rum is irresistible to the taste buds. There are a lot of healthy oats in these cookies as well.

A total of four dozen can be made from this recipe.

20 minutes of active time

40 minutes from start to finish

1 and a half cups of flaked unsweetened coconut

Gluten-free oat flour, 11.5 oz.

1-and-a-half cups of tapioca flour

2 tablespoons of oat bran

One and a half tablespoons of baking soda.

xanthan gum, 1 teaspoon

12 tsp. of salt

98   CHRISTMAS BASED GLUTEN-FREE RECIPES

Solidly packed light brown sugar, 1 1/2 cups

3 sticks of softened unsalted butter

Eggs of a large size

Rum extract: 1 tsp.

Three cups of gluten-free rolled oats.

Dried pineapple cubes

The oven should be preheated to 350°F. Using parchment paper or silicone baking mats, cover two baking sheets with the mixture. Using a baking sheet, spread out the coconut and bake it for 5 to 7 minutes, or until it's browned. Set aside for now.

Xanthan gum and salt can be used for the xanthan gum and baking soda in this recipe. Make a thorough stir.

In a third mixing bowl, combine brown sugar and butter and beat on low speed with an electric mixer.

Mixing with an electric device. Beat at high speed for 3 to 4 minutes, or until the mixture is light and fluffier. Beat in the eggs and rum extract for a minute, then remove from the mixer.

To make stiff dough, add dry ingredients one at a time while continuing to beat the butter mixture.

Coconut, oats, and pineapple are all mixed in.

PINA COLADA OATMEAL COOKIES   99

Dough should be dropped in 1-tablespoon portions onto the prepared baking sheets, with two baking sheets spare.

Balls are separated by a few inches. Use the bottom of a rice-flour-dusted glass to gently flatten the mounds.

A mild browning should be visible after 10 to 12 minutes of baking. Allow cookies to cool for two minutes on the baking sheets before transferring to a wire rack to finish cooling.

Variation

Dried pineapple can be replaced with raisins or chopped dried apricots, for example.

In this recipe, you may either use pre-made gluten-free oat flour or make your own by grinding oats in a coffee grinder. To get ready for 11/4

There are around 11/2 cups worth of uncooked rolled oats in one cup of flour. Process them in tiny batches to avoid overcrowding the grinder.

Chapter Seventeen

CHOOLATE CHIPS COOKIES

The most popular cookie flavor is now available in a gluten-free form.

Produces two to three dozen

15 minutes of active time

30 minutes from start to finish

A quarter of a cup of finely chopped walnuts

Eleven and a half pounds of brown rice flour

2 tablespoons of brown sugar

Cornstarch is 1/4 cup.

Baking soda

Zanthan gum is 1/2 teaspoon.

12 tsp. of salt

102 CHRISTMAS BASED GLUTEN-FREE RECIPES

It need about 12 tablespoons of softened unsalted butter (1/2 stick) 1 cup light brown sugar, tightly packed

Eggs of a large size

1 tsp. of pure vanilla essence

Bittersweet chocolate chips in a 12-ounce bag

The oven should be preheated to 350°F. Using parchment paper or silicone baking mats, cover two baking sheets with the mixture. For 5 to 7 minutes, roast walnuts on a baking sheet in the oven.

Pour the flours into a mixing bowl and mix thoroughly. 3. Add the baking soda and xanthan gum and mix thoroughly. 4. Add the salt and mix thoroughly. Make a thorough stir.

3. Use an electric mixer on low speed to combine the butter and sugar in a separate mixing basin. Beat at high speed for 3 to 4 minutes, or until the mixture is light and fluffier. Beat for a full minute after adding the eggs and vanilla.

To make stiff dough, add dry ingredients one at a time while continuing to beat the butter mixture.

Add the chopped walnuts and chocolate chips and mix until well combined.

Dough should be dropped in 1-tablespoon portions onto the prepared baking sheets, with two baking sheets spare.

CHOOLATE CHIPS COOKIES

inches of spacing between cookies.

A mild browning should be visible after 10 to 12 minutes of baking. Allow cookies to cool for two minutes on the baking sheets before transferring to a wire rack to finish cooling.

Variations

For a festive twist on these cookies, use red and green candy-coated chocolate chips instead of the regular chips.

Macadamia nuts can be used in place of walnuts, and white chocolate chips can be used instead of bittersweet.

Ruth Graves Wakefield, owner of the Toll House Inn in Whitman, Massachusetts, invented the chocolate chip cookie in 1930. In addition to its home-style meals, the restaurant's success was boosted by its owner's habit of giving customers an extra helping of their entrée and a plate of her handmade cookies for dessert.

Chapter Eighteen

CHOCO COOKIES FROM MEXICO

Cinnamon and ground almonds flavor Mexican chocolate brand Ibarra, which is offered in blocks and is commonly used to make hot chocolate. These cookies also have those flavor subtleties.

Amount Produced: Two dozen

20 minutes of active time

40 minutes from start to finish

Almonds blanched to a fine powder

Sugar, divided into three equal portions: 3 cups

Dutch-process cocoa powder is 3/4 cup

1 tsp. cinnamon powder

12 tsp. of salt

5 ounces of finely chopped bittersweet chocolate

Large, room-temperature 4 egg whites

106 CHRISTMAS BASED GLUTEN-FREE RECIPES

Pure almond extract in a half teaspoon

Set the oven to 350 degrees Fahrenheit and prepare the food. Using parchment paper or silicone baking mats, cover two baking sheets with the mixture. For 5 to 7 minutes, roast almonds on a baking sheet in the oven.

2. Reduce the oven temperature to 325°F. 3. Reduce the oven time to 20 minutes. 1 cup confectioners' sugar and almonds in a large bowl.

Process the sugar and almonds in a food processor fitted with a steel blade, pulsing on and off as necessary.

3. Add remaining sugar, cocoa powder, cinnamon, and salt to almond mixture in a mixing dish. Add the egg whites, chocolate, and almond essence and mix thoroughly. Stir thoroughly.

4. Scoop out 1-tablespoon amounts of dough and place them on the baking sheets, 2 at a time

inches apart A cookie should be dry after baking for 20 to 25 minutes. Cool treats.

cool for 2 minutes before transferring to a wire rack to complete the cooling process.

Variation

Walnuts and vanilla extract can be used in place of the almonds and the almond extract, respectively.

Remove the cinnamon from the recipe.

When the rainy season comes, a tropical evergreen tree's inner bark — known as cinnamon — is removed and allowed to dry. Sticks or ground are sold at that time. Ceylon cinnamon, which has a less strong flavor, can be substituted for cassia in recipes.

CPSIA information can be obtained
at www.ICGtesting.com
Printed in the USA
LVHW061207190722
723853LV00014B/553